Beyond Temptation: Navigating the Complexities of Sex Addiction

A Comprehensive Guide to Understanding, Treating, and Managing Sex Addiction

By

Evelyn Blackwood

Beyond Temptation

Catalog

Introduction

Defining Sex Addiction

Sex addiction is a condition that is characterized by compulsive and excessive sexual thoughts, fantasies, or behaviors that significantly impact an individual's daily functioning and well-being. In order for a person's sexual behaviors to be classified as addictive, they must meet the following criteria:

1. The behavior is recurrent and persistent; The individual repeatedly engages in sexual behavior, often despite negative consequences such as physical or emotional harm.

2. The behavior is out of control; The individual is unable to control their sexual thoughts, urges, or behaviors, often resulting in impulsivity and a lack of consideration for consequences.

3. The behavior is causing significant distress or impairment in social, occupational, or other important areas of functioning. The individual's sexual behaviors are interfering with their ability to function effectively in important aspects of their life, such as work, school, or relationships.

Sex addiction is often referred to as a process addiction, as it involves a pattern of behavior that provides a temporary sense of relief or pleasure, but ultimately leads to negative consequences. People with sex addiction may engage in a variety of sexual behaviors, including pornography use, anonymous sexual encounters, compulsive masturbation, or exhibitionism.

It's important to note that not all excessive or problematic sexual behaviors are indicative of sex addiction. It's normal for individuals to experience fluctuations in their sexual behavior and desire over time, and there is no one-size-fits-all definition of "normal" sexual behavior.

However, if an individual's sexual behaviors are causing significant distress or impairment in their life, it may be a sign of sex addiction and professional help may be needed.

Understanding the Stages of Sex Addiction

Sex addiction typically progresses through several stages, each of which can have a significant impact on an individual's life. While not all individuals with sex addiction will experience all of these stages, understanding the general progression of the condition can be helpful in recognizing when professional help may be needed.

1. **Preoccupation:** In the preoccupation stage, an individual becomes preoccupied with sexual thoughts, fantasies, or behaviors. They may spend an excessive amount of time thinking about sex, engaging in sexual behavior, or planning for future sexual encounters.

2. **Ritualization:** In the ritualization stage, an individual begins to develop a set of rituals or routines around their sexual behaviors. These rituals may include specific places, times of day, or types of sexual activity that they engage in.

3. **Compulsion:** In the compulsion stage, an individual begins to feel an intense urge to engage in sexual behavior, even if they know it will have negative consequences. They may feel as though they have no control over their sexual thoughts or behaviors.

4. **Despair:** In the despair stage, an individual begins to feel a sense of hopelessness and despair as they realize the negative impact that their sexual behaviors are having on their life. They may feel isolated, ashamed, and unable to seek help.

5. **Acting Out:** In the acting out stage, an individual begins to engage in more risky and dangerous sexual behaviors in order to achieve the same level of satisfaction or pleasure as before. This can lead to physical or emotional harm, as well as legal or financial consequences.

Understanding the stages of sex addiction can be helpful in recognizing when professional help may be needed. If you or someone you know is experiencing symptoms of sex addiction, it's important to seek help from a mental health professional who specializes in the treatment of sex addiction. Early intervention can help prevent the condition from progressing and can improve the chances of successful treatment and recovery.

Common Misconceptions about Sex Addiction

Sex addiction is a highly stigmatized condition, and there are many misconceptions about what it is and who it affects. Here are some common misconceptions about sex addiction:

1. **Sex addiction is a choice:** Many people believe that individuals with sex addiction choose to engage in their sexual behaviors, and that they could stop if they wanted to. However, sex addiction is a complex condition that involves changes in brain chemistry and reward pathways. Individuals with sex addiction often feel as though they have no control over their sexual thoughts and behaviors, and may struggle to stop even if they want to.

2. **Sex addiction is only about sex:** While sex addiction does involve compulsive and excessive sexual behaviors, it is often a symptom of underlying emotional or psychological issues. People with sex addiction may use sex as a way to cope with stress, anxiety, or depression, or to numb painful emotions.

3. **Only men can have sex addiction:** Sex addiction affects people of all genders and sexual orientations. However, due to cultural and societal norms around gender and sexuality, men may be more likely to seek treatment for sex addiction, while women may be more likely to keep their struggles with sex addiction a secret.

4. **Sex addiction is the same as having a high sex drive:** While individuals with sex addiction may have a higher sex drive than average, having a high sex drive does not necessarily mean that someone has sex addiction. Sex addiction involves a loss of control over sexual thoughts and behaviors, and negative consequences in important areas of functioning.

5. **Sex addiction can be cured with willpower alone:** While willpower can be an important component of recovery from sex addiction, it is not enough to cure the condition on its own. Sex addiction often requires professional help, such as therapy, medication, or support groups, in order to achieve successful recovery.

Understanding the common misconceptions about sex addiction can help individuals with the condition and their loved ones to seek appropriate help and support, and to reduce the shame and stigma that can be associated with sex addiction.

Part I: The Roots of Sex Addiction

Chapter 1

Understanding the Development of Sex Addiction

Understanding the Development of Sex Addiction focuses on exploring the various factors that can contribute to the development of sex addiction. The chapter begins by defining sex addiction and its impact on individuals and relationships. It then delves into the role of genetics and family history in the development of sex addiction, including the influence of genetic factors and epigenetics, as well as the impact of family dynamics and environment.

The chapter then explores the impact of childhood experiences on the development of sex addiction, including how early trauma and neglect can contribute to the development of sex addiction. It also examines the connection between early sexual experiences and the development of sex addiction, including the role of sexual abuse, exploitation, or exposure, as well as the impact of early sexual experiences and pornography use.

The importance of a comprehensive assessment in understanding the development of sex addiction is also highlighted, including the role of mental health professionals in assessing and identifying contributing factors. Additionally, the chapter stresses the importance of considering co-occurring disorders and environmental factors in assessment.

Overall, Chapter 1 emphasizes the complex nature of the factors that can contribute to the development of sex addiction. By understanding these factors, individuals with sex addiction and mental health professionals can better develop effective treatment and recovery plans.

The influence of genetics and epigenetics on the development of sex addiction

The influence of genetics and epigenetics on the development of sex addiction is an important area of study in the field of addiction. Research has suggested that genetic factors may contribute to a predisposition towards addictive behaviors, including sex addiction.

For example, studies have found that certain genes involved in reward and impulse control, such as the dopamine receptor gene, may be associated with an increased risk of addictive behaviors. Additionally, epigenetic factors, which are modifications to genes that can be influenced by environmental factors, may also play a role in the development of sex addiction.

While genetics and epigenetics are important areas of study, it is important to note that they do not solely determine the development of sex addiction. Environmental factors, such as childhood experiences and social and cultural influences, also play a significant role.

Ultimately, understanding the role of genetics and epigenetics in sex addiction can help individuals and mental health professionals develop more effective prevention and treatment strategies for the disorder.

The impact of family history and environment on the development of sex addiction

The impact of family history and environment on the development of sex addiction is another important area of study in understanding the roots of the disorder. Research has suggested that family dynamics and environmental factors can contribute to the development of sex addiction.

Individuals who grew up in families with a history of addiction or dysfunctional family dynamics may be more likely to develop sex addiction. This can be due to a combination of genetic and environmental factors, including a higher risk of exposure to addiction, neglect, or trauma.

Social and cultural influences can also impact the development of sex addiction. In a culture that often promotes and glamorizes sexual behavior, individuals may feel pressure to engage in risky sexual behavior or view pornography. This can lead to the development of a sex addiction.

Understanding the impact of family history and environment on the development of sex addiction can help individuals and mental health professionals develop more effective prevention and treatment strategies for the disorder. This can include addressing underlying family dynamics and trauma, as well as promoting healthy coping strategies and social support networks.

How to identify and address genetic and familial factors in the treatment of sex addiction

Identifying and addressing genetic and familial factors in the treatment of sex addiction can be a challenging but important part of recovery. Here are some strategies that can help:

1. **Family history assessment:** Conducting a thorough assessment of the client's family history of addiction, mental health issues, and other relevant factors can provide valuable information on the potential genetic and familial risk factors for sex addiction.

2. **Psychological evaluation:** A psychological evaluation can help identify underlying emotional and psychological issues that may contribute to sex addiction. This can include issues such as depression, anxiety, trauma, or attachment disorders.

3. **Family therapy:** Family therapy can be a helpful tool in addressing family dynamics and communication patterns that may contribute to sex addiction. This can involve working with the client's family to address issues such as addiction, codependency, or dysfunction.

4. **Genetic testing:** Genetic testing can provide valuable information on potential genetic risk factors for addiction. While this is not currently a routine part of treatment, it may be considered in certain cases.

5. **Collaborative care:** Collaborative care involving a multidisciplinary team, including mental health professionals, medical providers, and addiction specialists, can help address the complex needs of individuals with sex addiction and provide more effective treatment.

Ultimately, identifying and addressing genetic and familial factors in the treatment of sex addiction can help individuals achieve long-term recovery and lead fulfilling, healthy lives.

Chapter 2

Early Life Experiences and Trauma in the Development of Sex Addiction

Early life experiences and trauma can also play a significant role in the development of sex addiction. Trauma, neglect, or abuse during childhood can lead to a range of emotional, psychological, and behavioral issues, including sex addiction.

Studies have found that individuals who experience childhood trauma, such as sexual abuse, physical abuse, or neglect, are at higher risk of developing sex addiction. This may be due to a number of factors, including the development of maladaptive coping strategies, low self-esteem, and difficulty with emotional regulation.

Early experiences of sexualization or exposure to pornography can also impact the development of sex addiction. For example, individuals who were exposed to pornography at a young age may develop a distorted view of sex and intimacy, leading to problematic sexual behavior later in life.

Understanding the impact of early life experiences and trauma on the development of sex addiction is crucial in developing effective treatment strategies. This can include addressing underlying trauma, promoting healthy coping mechanisms, and developing healthy relationships with others.

Treatment for sex addiction may involve a combination of therapy, support groups, and medication to address underlying psychological issues and promote healthy coping mechanisms. Additionally, self-care practices such as exercise, meditation, and journaling can also be helpful in promoting emotional and psychological well-being.

Overall, understanding the role of early life experiences and trauma in the development of sex addiction can provide valuable insights into the disorder and guide effective treatment strategies for individuals struggling with this issue.

The role of early life experiences in the development of sex addiction

Early life experiences can play a significant role in the development of sex addiction. Children who grow up in environments where sex is not openly discussed or who receive negative messages about sex may develop unhealthy attitudes or behaviors around sexuality. For example, children who receive inadequate or overly harsh sexual education may develop feelings of shame or guilt around their own sexual desires, leading to compulsive and secretive behaviors later in life.

Individuals who experience neglect or abuse during childhood may also be at higher risk for developing sex addiction. This may be due to a number of factors, including the development of maladaptive coping strategies, low self-esteem, and difficulty with emotional regulation.

Research has also shown that early experiences of sexualization or exposure to pornography can impact the development of sex addiction. For example, individuals who were exposed to pornography at a young age may develop a distorted view of sex and intimacy, leading to problematic sexual behavior later in life.

Understanding the role of early life experiences in the development of sex addiction is important for developing effective treatment strategies. This can include addressing underlying trauma, promoting healthy coping mechanisms, and developing healthy relationships with others.

Treatment for sex addiction may involve a combination of therapy, support groups, and medication to address underlying psychological issues and promote healthy coping mechanisms. Additionally, self-care practices such as exercise, meditation, and journaling can also be helpful in promoting emotional and psychological well-being.

Overall, recognizing the impact of early life experiences on the development of sex addiction can provide valuable insights into the disorder and guide effective treatment strategies for individuals struggling with this issue.

The impact of childhood trauma and neglect on the development of sex addiction

Childhood trauma and neglect can have a profound impact on an individual's emotional and psychological development, which can in turn contribute to the development of sex addiction. When children experience neglect or abuse, they may develop maladaptive coping mechanisms such as addictive behaviors to cope with emotional pain and distress.

For example, children who have experienced sexual abuse or other forms of trauma may turn to sex addiction as a way to cope with feelings of shame, guilt, and low self-esteem. Additionally, individuals who have experienced neglect or emotional abuse may struggle with intimacy and emotional connection, leading them to seek out sexual experiences as a way to feel validated and connected with others.

It is important to note that not all individuals who experience childhood trauma or neglect will develop sex addiction. However, the impact of childhood experiences should be considered in assessment and treatment of the disorder.

By addressing the underlying emotional and psychological factors that contribute to sex addiction, individuals can develop healthier coping mechanisms and reduce the risk of relapse.

How to address early life experiences and trauma in the treatment of sex addiction

Addressing early life experiences and trauma is an important aspect of treating sex addiction. It is important for mental health professionals to create a safe and supportive environment in which clients can explore and process their past experiences.

One approach to addressing early life experiences and trauma is through individual therapy, such as cognitive-behavioral therapy (CBT) or trauma-focused therapy. These therapies can help clients identify and address maladaptive coping mechanisms, negative thought patterns, and emotional triggers that contribute to sex addiction.

In addition to individual therapy, group therapy and support groups can also be effective in addressing early life experiences and trauma. Group therapy allows clients to connect with others who have had similar experiences, and provides a supportive environment for exploring and processing emotions.

It is also important for mental health professionals to address any co-occurring mental health disorders, such as depression or anxiety, that may be contributing to sex addiction. This may involve medication management and other forms of psychotherapy.

Ultimately, addressing early life experiences and trauma is an important aspect of treating sex addiction, and can help individuals develop healthier coping mechanisms.

Chapter 3

The Role of Psychological Factors in Sex Addiction

Chapter 3 explores the role of psychological factors in sex addiction. While early life experiences and trauma can play a significant role in the development of sex addiction, there are also a number of psychological factors that can contribute to the disorder.

One such factor is attachment theory, which suggests that individuals who have insecure attachment styles may be more likely to develop sex addiction as a way of coping with emotional distress and seeking out validation and connection. Individuals with insecure attachment styles may struggle with intimacy and emotional connection, leading them to seek out sexual experiences as a way to feel validated and connected with others.

Other psychological factors that may contribute to sex addiction include personality traits such as impulsivity, sensation seeking, and low self-esteem. These traits can make individuals more vulnerable to addictive behaviors, and can contribute to the development of sex addiction.

In addition to individual factors, social and cultural factors may also contribute to sex addiction. For example, the prevalence of hypersexualized media and cultural messages about sex may contribute to the normalization of excessive sexual behavior and contribute to the development of sex addiction.

By understanding the role of psychological factors in sex addiction, mental health professionals can develop more effective treatment strategies that address the underlying emotional and psychological issues that contribute to the disorder.

Understanding the psychological factors that contribute to the development of sex addiction

Personality traits such as impulsivity, low self-esteem, and sensation seeking can make individuals more vulnerable to addictive behaviors, including sex addiction. These traits may contribute to the development of sex addiction by making individuals more likely to engage in risky sexual behaviors, and less able to regulate their sexual behavior.

Coping mechanisms and emotional regulation difficulties can also contribute to the development of sex addiction. Individuals who have difficulty managing their emotions may turn to sex as a way of coping with stress, anxiety, or other negative emotions. This can lead to a pattern of compulsive sexual behavior, as individuals become reliant on sex as a way of regulating their emotions.

It is important for mental health professionals to identify and address these psychological factors in the treatment of sex addiction. Cognitive-behavioral therapy (CBT) and other forms of psychotherapy can be effective in helping individuals develop healthier coping mechanisms and emotional regulation strategies. In addition, mindfulness-based approaches and other holistic therapies can help individuals develop greater self-awareness and learn to regulate their emotions in healthier ways.

Ultimately, by understanding the psychological factors that contribute to the development of sex addiction, mental health professionals can develop more effective treatment strategies that address the underlying emotional and psychological issues that contribute to the disorder.

The impact of cognitive distortions on individuals with sex addiction

Cognitive distortions are patterns of thinking that are irrational or inaccurate, and that can lead to negative emotional and behavioral outcomes.

In the context of sex addiction, individuals may experience cognitive distortions related to their sexual behavior, such as beliefs that they cannot control their sexual urges, that their sexual behavior is normal or harmless, or that their behavior is necessary for their well-being or self-worth. These cognitive distortions can contribute to the development and maintenance of sex addiction, as individuals may use these beliefs to justify their compulsive sexual behavior and avoid seeking help.

Addressing cognitive distortions is an important part of the treatment of sex addiction. Cognitive-behavioral therapy (CBT) is an effective treatment approach that focuses on identifying and challenging these distorted beliefs, and replacing them with more rational and accurate thoughts. This can help individuals develop healthier attitudes and beliefs about sex, and reduce the frequency and intensity of their compulsive sexual behavior.

In addition to CBT, mindfulness-based approaches and other forms of psychotherapy can also be effective in helping individuals with sex addiction develop greater self-awareness and identify and address their cognitive distortions. By addressing these cognitive distortions, individuals with sex addiction can gain greater insight into their behavior and develop healthier attitudes and beliefs about sex.

How to address psychological factors in the treatment of sex addiction

In addressing psychological factors in the treatment of sex addiction, it is important to understand the underlying causes and triggers of the behavior. As discussed earlier, personality traits, coping mechanisms, and emotional regulation difficulties can all contribute to the development of sex addiction. Therefore, an effective treatment approach should focus on addressing these factors.

Cognitive-behavioral therapy (CBT) is one effective approach that can be used to address psychological factors in the treatment of sex addiction. This therapy aims to help individuals identify and challenge their negative or distorted beliefs and thought patterns, and replace them with more rational and healthy ones. CBT can also help individuals learn new coping skills and strategies to manage their emotions and behaviors.

Another effective approach is psychodynamic therapy, which aims to help individuals explore and understand the unconscious motives and conflicts that may be driving their sexual behavior. Through this process of self-exploration and reflection, individuals can gain a greater understanding of their behavior and develop new ways of coping and relating to others.

Other techniques that can be used to address psychological factors in the treatment of sex addiction include mindfulness-based therapies, group therapy, and family therapy. The most effective treatment approach will depend on the individual's unique needs and circumstances, and may involve a combination of different therapies and techniques.

Chapter 4

The Connection between Attachment and Sex Addiction

Chapter 4 explores the connection between attachment and sex addiction. Attachment theory posits that early attachment experiences with caregivers shape an individual's attachment style, which in turn influences their relationships and behaviors later in life. Research has shown that insecure attachment styles are associated with a higher risk for a range of mental health issues, including addiction.

In the context of sex addiction, insecure attachment styles may contribute to a lack of emotional intimacy and a reliance on sexual experiences to fulfill emotional needs. Individuals with insecure attachment may struggle with intimacy, communication, and emotional regulation, which can lead to a reliance on sexual experiences to feel validated and connected.

Understanding the role of attachment in sex addiction can be helpful in developing effective treatment approaches. Treatment may focus on helping individuals develop secure attachment styles and learn healthy ways of relating to others. This may involve exploring past attachment experiences and working to develop more positive relationships and attachment patterns. Techniques such as attachment-based therapy and experiential therapy may be useful in addressing attachment issues in the context of sex addiction.

Understanding attachment theory and its connection to sex addiction

Attachment theory is a psychological theory that explains how early attachment experiences with primary caregivers shape an individual's attachment style and influence their relationships and behaviors later in life. According to attachment theory, individuals develop either a secure or an insecure attachment style based on their experiences with caregivers during their formative years.

In the context of sex addiction, insecure attachment styles are thought to contribute to a reliance on sexual experiences to fulfill emotional needs. For example, individuals with an anxious attachment style may have a strong need for intimacy and connection but may struggle with trust and fear of abandonment. This may lead them to engage in compulsive sexual behaviors as a way to seek validation and reassurance from others. Individuals with an avoidant attachment style, on the other hand, may struggle with emotional intimacy and may use sex as a way to avoid closeness and emotional vulnerability.

Understanding the connection between attachment and sex addiction can be helpful in developing effective treatment approaches. Treatment may focus on helping individuals develop secure attachment styles and learn healthy ways of relating to others. This may involve exploring past attachment experiences and working to develop more positive relationships and attachment patterns. Techniques such as attachment-based therapy and experiential therapy may be useful in addressing attachment issues in the context of sex addiction.

The impact of insecure attachment styles on the development of sex addiction

Insecure attachment styles can have a significant impact on the development of sex addiction. Individuals with insecure attachment styles may struggle with emotional regulation and experience difficulty in forming healthy relationships, which can lead them to rely on sexual experiences to fulfill their emotional needs.

For example, individuals with an anxious attachment style may feel a constant need for intimacy and connection but may also experience fear of abandonment and rejection. They may turn to sex and sexual fantasies as a way to cope with these emotions and seek validation and reassurance from others. This can lead to compulsive sexual behaviors and addiction.

Similarly, individuals with an avoidant attachment style may struggle with emotional intimacy and vulnerability. They may use sex as a way to avoid closeness and emotional connection with others. This can also lead to compulsive sexual behaviors and addiction.

Overall, the impact of insecure attachment styles on the development of sex addiction highlights the importance of addressing attachment issues in the treatment of sex addiction. Treatment may involve exploring past attachment experiences, working to develop more positive relationships and attachment patterns, and addressing emotional regulation difficulties.

How therapy can help individuals with sex addiction to develop more secure attachment styles

Therapy can be an effective tool for individuals with sex addiction to develop more secure attachment styles. One approach is to work with a therapist to identify patterns in their attachment style and understand how these patterns are impacting their sexual behaviors and addiction.

The therapist may also help the individual to explore any unresolved attachment-related issues from their past, such as childhood trauma, neglect, or abuse. By understanding and processing these past experiences, individuals can begin to develop healthier attachment patterns and learn to regulate their emotions in a more effective way.

In addition, therapy can provide individuals with skills and strategies to develop more positive and fulfilling relationships with others. For example, the therapist may work with the individual to improve communication skills, increase emotional awareness and empathy, and develop more effective coping mechanisms.

Overall, therapy can be a crucial component of addressing attachment issues in the treatment of sex addiction, helping individuals to develop more secure attachment styles and improve their emotional well-being.

Chapter 5

The Connection between Shame and Sex Addiction

Shame is a complex emotion that can have a significant impact on individuals struggling with sex addiction. Chapter 5 explores the connection between shame and sex addiction, including how shame can contribute to the development and maintenance of sex addiction.

The chapter also examines the role of shame in perpetuating the cycle of sex addiction, as individuals may engage in sexual behaviors as a way to cope with or avoid feelings of shame. This can lead to a vicious cycle in which shame and sex addiction feed into each other.

Finally, the chapter discusses how to address shame in the treatment of sex addiction. Therapies such as cognitive-behavioral therapy (CBT), mindfulness-based interventions, and group therapy can be effective in helping individuals to identify and challenge their negative beliefs about themselves and their sexual behaviors. By reducing shame, individuals can begin to break free from the cycle of sex addiction and develop a more positive sense of self.

The role of shame in the development and maintenance of sex addiction

Shame can play a significant role in the development and maintenance of sex addiction. Individuals with sex addiction often experience intense feelings of shame and guilt associated with their sexual behaviors, which can contribute to a cycle of addiction.

Shame can lead individuals to engage in secretive and isolating behaviors, such as hiding their sexual behaviors from others or avoiding social situations. This can further exacerbate feelings of shame and lead to a sense of loneliness and disconnection from others.

Additionally, individuals with sex addiction may use sexual behaviors as a way to cope with or avoid feelings of shame. This can create a self-perpetuating cycle, in which the sexual behaviors lead to more shame and the shame leads to more sexual behaviors.

It's important to address the role of shame in the treatment of sex addiction. Therapies such as cognitive-behavioral therapy (CBT) and mindfulness-based interventions can be effective in helping individuals to identify and challenge their negative beliefs about themselves and their sexual behaviors. Group therapy can also be helpful in providing a supportive and non-judgmental environment for individuals to share their experiences and feelings of shame.

By reducing shame, individuals can begin to break free from the cycle of sex addiction and develop a more positive sense of self.

The impact of internalized shame on individuals with sex addiction

Internalized shame can have a profound impact on individuals with sex addiction. Shame can lead individuals to feel unworthy, unlovable, and inherently flawed, which can contribute to feelings of depression, anxiety, and low self-esteem. Internalized shame can also lead to self-destructive behaviors, such as substance abuse or self-harm.

For individuals with sex addiction, internalized shame can lead to a cycle of addiction. The shame associated with their sexual behaviors can lead to feelings of distress and the need for relief, which can then lead to engaging in more sexual behaviors. This can create a vicious cycle, in which the shame associated with the behaviors leads to more behaviors, and the behaviors lead to more shame.

It's important to address internalized shame in the treatment of sex addiction. Therapies such as cognitive-behavioral therapy (CBT) and acceptance and commitment therapy (ACT) can be helpful in helping individuals to identify and challenge their negative beliefs about themselves and their sexual behaviors. Group therapy and support groups can also be helpful in providing a supportive and non-judgmental environment for individuals to share their experiences and feelings of shame. By reducing internalized shame, individuals can begin to break free from the cycle of sex addiction and develop a more positive sense of self.

How to address shame in the treatment of sex addiction

Addressing shame in the treatment of sex addiction can be a complex process, but there are several approaches that can be helpful. Some of these approaches include:

1. **Identifying the source of shame:** It can be helpful to explore the underlying beliefs and experiences that contribute to the individual's feelings of shame. This may involve identifying early childhood experiences or cultural messages that have contributed to their shame.

2. **Challenging negative beliefs:** Cognitive-behavioral therapy (CBT) can be helpful in addressing negative thoughts and beliefs that contribute to feelings of shame. Through CBT, individuals can learn to challenge their negative thoughts and develop more positive self-talk.

3. **Mindfulness and acceptance-based approaches:** Acceptance and commitment therapy (ACT) and other mindfulness-based approaches can be helpful in teaching individuals to be more accepting and non-judgmental of their experiences, including their feelings of shame.

4. **Group therapy and support groups:** Group therapy and support groups can be helpful in providing a supportive and non-judgmental environment for individuals to share their experiences and feelings of shame. By connecting with others who have similar experiences, individuals can feel less alone and more understood.

5. **Developing a sense of self-compassion:** Developing a sense of self-compassion can be helpful in reducing feelings of shame. Through self-compassion practices, individuals can learn to be kinder and more understanding of themselves, which can help to reduce feelings of shame and self-criticism.

By addressing shame in the treatment of sex addiction, individuals can begin to break free from the cycle of addiction and develop a more positive sense of self.

Part II: The Impact of Sex Addiction

Chapter 1

Emotional Dysregulation in Sex Addiction

Emotional dysregulation refers to the inability to manage or regulate one's emotions effectively. In the context of sex addiction, emotional dysregulation can play a significant role in both the development and maintenance of the addiction. Individuals with sex addiction may use sexual behavior as a way to cope with difficult emotions, such as anxiety, depression, shame, or loneliness. However, engaging in sexual behaviors can create a cycle of shame and guilt, which further reinforces emotional dysregulation and perpetuates the addiction. This can lead to a range of negative emotional consequences, such as feelings of emptiness, low self-esteem, and a sense of being out of control.

The link between emotional dysregulation and other psychological conditions, such as anxiety and depression

Emotional dysregulation is commonly associated with other psychological conditions, such as anxiety and depression. When emotions are not managed effectively, they can intensify and lead to symptoms of anxiety or depression. For example, individuals with sex addiction may feel anxious or depressed when they are unable to engage in sexual behavior, or they may experience a sense of emptiness or depression after engaging in sexual behavior. This can create a cycle of negative emotions and behaviors that can be difficult to break without proper treatment. Addressing emotional dysregulation in the treatment of sex addiction can be important for improving overall mental health and reducing symptoms of anxiety and depression.

How emotional dysregulation affects interpersonal relationships and overall quality of life

Emotional dysregulation can have a significant impact on interpersonal relationships and overall quality of life for individuals with sex addiction. When emotions are not managed effectively, it can lead to impulsive or risky behavior that can damage relationships with partners, family, and friends. This can lead to feelings of isolation, loneliness, and shame. Additionally, the focus on sexual behavior can interfere with work, school, and other important aspects of daily life, leading to further stress and anxiety. Addressing emotional dysregulation in the treatment of sex addiction can improve overall functioning, increase feelings of connection with others, and enhance quality of life.

Chapter 2

Shame and Guilt in Sex Addiction

Shame and guilt are common emotions experienced by individuals with sex addiction, and they can have a significant impact on their mental health and well-being. Shame can lead to feelings of worthlessness, self-hatred, and a sense of being fundamentally flawed. Guilt, on the other hand, is a response to specific behaviors and actions, and can lead to a focus on the negative consequences of those behaviors. Both shame and guilt can interfere with the ability to form healthy relationships, can lead to a preoccupation with sexual behavior, and can exacerbate emotional dysregulation. Addressing shame and guilt in the treatment of sex addiction can help individuals to work through these difficult emotions, increase their self-esteem, and develop more healthy coping strategies.

The relationship between shame, guilt, and relapse

Shame and guilt are commonly experienced by individuals with sex addiction, and they can play a significant role in triggering relapse. Feelings of shame may arise from the fear of being caught or exposed, while guilt may stem from the realization of the harm caused to oneself or others. These emotions can lead to a cycle of negative self-talk, self-blame, and increased stress, which can increase the risk of relapse.

Furthermore, relapse can further intensify feelings of shame and guilt, creating a vicious cycle that can be difficult to break. This is why it is essential to address shame and guilt in the treatment of sex addiction, to help individuals develop healthier coping mechanisms and improve their overall emotional well-being.

Strategies for addressing shame and guilt in therapy

There are several strategies that can be used to address shame and guilt in therapy for individuals with sex addiction. One approach is to help individuals identify and challenge the irrational thoughts and beliefs that contribute to their feelings of shame and guilt. This may involve cognitive-behavioral techniques, such as cognitive restructuring or exposure therapy.

Another strategy is to help individuals develop self-compassion and acceptance. This can involve mindfulness practices, such as meditation or breathing exercises, as well as psychoeducation about the common humanity of addiction and the need for self-forgiveness.

Family therapy and couples therapy can also be helpful in addressing the impact of shame and guilt on interpersonal relationships. Family members can learn to provide support and validation while also setting appropriate boundaries and expectations for behavior.

Chapter 3

Trauma and Post-Traumatic Stress Disorder (PTSD) in Sex Addiction

Sex addiction can be closely linked to trauma and post-traumatic stress disorder (PTSD). Trauma can be defined as an event or experience that is outside the realm of normal human experience and overwhelms an individual's ability to cope with the situation. Trauma can take many forms, such as sexual abuse, physical abuse, emotional abuse, neglect, and other experiences that are physically or emotionally threatening.

PTSD is a mental health condition that can develop in people who have experienced or witnessed a traumatic event. Symptoms of PTSD can include intrusive thoughts, nightmares, flashbacks, avoidance behavior, and hyperarousal. Individuals with sex addiction may experience symptoms of PTSD related to their sexual behaviors, such as intrusive thoughts about sexual acts or images, anxiety related to sexual experiences, and avoidance of sexual situations.

Trauma and PTSD can contribute to the development of sex addiction by creating a need for coping mechanisms and a desire to escape from painful emotions. Individuals with trauma histories may turn to sex addiction as a way to numb or distract themselves from difficult feelings. Additionally, traumatic experiences can lead to a sense of powerlessness or a desire for control, which can manifest in sexual behaviors.

It's important for therapists to recognize the connection between trauma, PTSD, and sex addiction in order to provide effective treatment. Trauma-informed therapy approaches, such as EMDR (eye movement desensitization and reprocessing), can be helpful in addressing the underlying trauma that may be contributing to sex addiction. Additionally, mindfulness-based interventions and other coping strategies can help individuals learn to regulate their emotions and reduce the need for maladaptive coping mechanisms like sex addiction.

How individuals with a history of trauma may use sex addiction as a coping mechanism

Individuals who have experienced trauma may struggle with a range of emotional difficulties such as anxiety, depression, and PTSD, which can make them more vulnerable to addiction. Trauma can lead to a sense of powerlessness, and for some individuals, sex addiction can become a way to feel in control or numb painful emotions. In addition, trauma can lead to feelings of shame, guilt, and low self-esteem, which can reinforce a cycle of addictive behavior. As a coping mechanism, sex addiction may provide temporary relief, but ultimately, it can exacerbate existing emotional difficulties and prevent individuals from engaging in healthy coping strategies.

The role of trauma-focused therapy in the treatment of sex addiction

Trauma-focused therapy can be an effective treatment approach for individuals with sex addiction who have a history of trauma. This type of therapy aims to help individuals process and work through traumatic experiences in a safe and supportive environment.

Techniques such as cognitive processing therapy, eye movement desensitization and reprocessing (EMDR), and prolonged exposure therapy can be used to address traumatic memories and reduce the symptoms of PTSD. By addressing the underlying trauma that may have contributed to the development of sex addiction, individuals can begin to develop healthier coping mechanisms and reduce their reliance on addictive behaviors.

Chapter 4

Intimacy Issues in Sex Addiction

Sex addiction can greatly impact an individual's ability to form and maintain intimate relationships. Individuals with sex addiction may experience difficulty with emotional intimacy, may struggle to communicate their needs and desires, and may have difficulty establishing healthy boundaries in relationships. Additionally, sex addiction can lead to infidelity, which can cause significant damage to a relationship. Over time, the impact of sex addiction on an individual's relationships can lead to feelings of loneliness, isolation, and a sense of disconnection from others. Addressing sex addiction through therapy can help individuals learn healthier relationship skills and establish fulfilling, meaningful connections with others.

The effects of sex addiction on trust, vulnerability, and emotional intimacy

Sex addiction can have a significant impact on an individual's ability to form and maintain intimate relationships. Trust is a crucial component of any relationship, and the secrecy and shame surrounding sex addiction can erode trust between partners. Individuals with sex addiction may struggle with vulnerability, as they may fear being judged or rejected by their partners if their addiction is revealed. This fear can lead to emotional distance and a lack of intimacy in the relationship.

Moreover, sex addiction can create a sense of emotional disconnection, as the focus is often on the physical act of sex rather than emotional connection. Individuals with sex addiction may use sex as a way to avoid emotional intimacy and may struggle with expressing their emotions in a healthy way.

Additionally, the consequences of sex addiction, such as infidelity or sexual boundary violations, can cause significant emotional harm to partners, leading to feelings of betrayal, hurt, and anger. It is essential for individuals with sex addiction to seek treatment not only for their own well-being but also for the health of their relationships.

Strategies for addressing intimacy issues in therapy for sex addiction.

There are several strategies that can be employed in therapy to address intimacy issues in individuals with sex addiction. One approach is to focus on building healthy communication skills and encouraging the individual to express their feelings and needs openly with their partner. Additionally, therapists may use techniques such as cognitive-behavioral therapy (CBT) to challenge negative thought patterns and beliefs about intimacy and relationships.

Another strategy is to encourage the individual to practice mindfulness and self-compassion, which can help them to become more comfortable with vulnerability and emotional intimacy. This may involve teaching the individual techniques such as meditation or deep breathing exercises to help them manage their emotions and stay present in the moment.

It may also be helpful to involve the partner in therapy to work on building trust and addressing any issues in the relationship that may be contributing to the individual's sex addiction. Couples therapy can be an effective way to improve communication, build intimacy, and develop a deeper understanding of each other's needs and desires.

Relationship Issues and Sex Addiction

Individuals struggling with sex addiction often face significant relationship issues, including infidelity, dishonesty, and communication difficulties. These issues can arise in various types of relationships, including romantic partnerships, friendships, and familial relationships.

One of the primary challenges for individuals with sex addiction is maintaining healthy boundaries in relationships. They may struggle to form intimate connections without seeking out sexual gratification, leading to cycles of destructive behavior that can damage relationships.

In addition, sex addiction can create a significant strain on existing relationships, leading to feelings of betrayal, anger, and mistrust. These issues can be especially challenging to navigate for partners of individuals with sex addiction, who may feel confused or overwhelmed by their loved one's behavior.

It is essential for individuals with sex addiction to address relationship issues in therapy to improve their ability to form healthy, intimate connections. Therapy can help individuals learn effective communication skills, establish and maintain boundaries, and develop healthy coping mechanisms for managing the challenges of intimate relationships.

Physical and Health Consequences of Sex Addiction

Sex addiction can have significant physical and health consequences. Individuals with sex addiction may engage in high-risk sexual behavior, such as having unprotected sex or engaging in sexual activities with multiple partners, which can increase the risk of contracting sexually transmitted infections (STIs). In addition, excessive sexual activity can lead to physical exhaustion and depletion, as well as injuries such as genital injuries or repetitive strain injuries.

Individuals with sex addiction may also experience physical health consequences as a result of co-occurring substance use disorders or other addictive behaviors, such as compulsive overeating or gambling. Substance use can lead to a range of physical health problems, including liver damage, cardiovascular disease, and respiratory problems.

Moreover, sex addiction can also have a negative impact on an individual's mental health, which in turn can affect their physical health. For example, depression and anxiety, which are commonly associated with sex addiction, can lead to a range of physical symptoms, such as fatigue, headaches, and muscle pain. Additionally, sex addiction may also result in sleep disturbances, which can contribute to a range of physical health problems, including obesity, diabetes, and heart disease.

It is important for individuals with sex addiction to address the physical and health consequences of their behavior in therapy. This may involve medical treatment for STIs or other physical health problems, as well as support and guidance to adopt healthy lifestyle habits and manage any co-occurring substance use or mental health disorders.

Part III: Treatment and Recovery

Sex addiction is a complex and challenging condition to treat, but there are many effective treatment options available. The goal of treatment is to help individuals overcome their compulsive sexual behavior and learn healthy coping mechanisms and strategies to manage triggers and prevent relapse.

Types of Treatment for Sex Addiction

There are several types of treatment for sex addiction. Some of the most common include:

1. **Individual therapy:** This type of therapy involves one-on-one sessions with a trained therapist. The therapist may use a variety of techniques, such as cognitive-behavioral therapy (CBT), psychodynamic therapy, or trauma-focused therapy, to help the individual understand the root causes of their addiction and develop coping skills to manage their behaviors.

2. **Group therapy:** Group therapy involves sessions with a therapist and other individuals who are struggling with sex addiction. The group provides a supportive environment where members can share their experiences, learn from one another, and offer each other encouragement and support.

3. **Couples therapy:** Couples therapy can be beneficial for individuals who are in a committed relationship and want to work on their addiction together. The therapist can help both partners understand the impact of the addiction on the relationship and develop strategies to rebuild trust and intimacy.

4. **Residential treatment:** Residential treatment involves living in a specialized facility for a period of time, typically 30 to 90 days. This type of treatment provides a structured and intensive program that includes individual and group therapy, educational classes, and other activities designed to promote healing and recovery.

5. **12-Step programs:** 12-Step programs, such as Sex Addicts Anonymous (SAA) or Sex and Love Addicts Anonymous (SLAA), are based on a spiritual approach to recovery and involve attending meetings, working with a sponsor, and following a set of principles aimed at helping individuals maintain abstinence and achieve lasting recovery.

It's important to note that not all treatment options will work for everyone, and it may take some trial and error to find the right approach. It's also important for individuals with sex addiction to work with a qualified therapist or treatment provider who has experience working with this specific issue.

Developing a Relapse Prevention Plan

Developing a relapse prevention plan is an important component of treatment and recovery for sex addiction. A relapse prevention plan is a personalized strategy that individuals can use to identify and avoid triggers and manage cravings and urges.

The first step in developing a relapse prevention plan is to identify triggers or situations that can lead to relapse. Triggers can include stress, anxiety, boredom, exposure to sexual content, or feelings of loneliness or rejection. Once triggers are identified, individuals can develop strategies to avoid or cope with them. For example, if exposure to sexual content is a trigger, individuals can limit their access to pornography or avoid certain websites or social media platforms.

The next step is to develop coping strategies to manage cravings and urges. Coping strategies can include relaxation techniques, such as deep breathing or mindfulness meditation, engaging in physical activity, or distracting oneself with hobbies or other activities.

It is also important to have a support system in place. This can include a therapist or support group, as well as family and friends who can provide encouragement and accountability.

Finally, it is important to review and adjust the relapse prevention plan regularly. As individuals progress in their recovery, triggers and coping strategies may change, so it is important to stay aware of these changes and adjust the plan accordingly.

Support Networks and Resources

Support networks and resources are essential for individuals seeking treatment and recovery from sex addiction. They provide a sense of community, understanding, and encouragement during the recovery process. There are various types of support networks and resources available, including:

1. **Support groups:** These are groups of individuals who have experienced or are experiencing similar issues with sex addiction. They meet regularly to provide emotional support, share experiences, and offer advice to each other.

2. **Therapy:** Therapy is a crucial component of treatment for sex addiction. A trained therapist can help individuals identify underlying issues, develop coping skills, and work towards recovery.

3. **12-step programs:** 12-step programs, such as Sex Addicts Anonymous (SAA) and Sex and Love Addicts Anonymous (SLAA), provide a structured approach to recovery. They follow a set of principles that help individuals achieve sobriety and maintain long-term recovery.

4. **Online resources:** There are numerous online resources available for individuals seeking information and support for sex addiction. These include online support groups, educational materials, and forums.

5. **Professional organizations:** Professional organizations, such as the Society for the Advancement of Sexual Health (SASH) and the International Institute for Trauma and Addiction Professionals (IITAP), provide information and resources for professionals and individuals seeking help for sex addiction.

It's important to note that support networks and resources are not one-size-fits-all. What works for one individual may not work for another. It's essential to find the right support network and resources that suit an individual's unique needs and circumstances.

Part IV: Beyond Recovery

Rebuilding Relationships After Sex Addiction

Rebuilding relationships after sex addiction can be a long and challenging process. The impact of sex addiction on relationships can be devastating, leading to a breakdown of trust, communication, and emotional intimacy. However, with commitment and effort from both partners, it is possible to rebuild and strengthen the relationship.

One important aspect of rebuilding a relationship after sex addiction is to establish open and honest communication. Both partners should be willing to talk openly and honestly about their feelings, fears, and concerns. This can help to rebuild trust and create a deeper emotional connection between the partners.

Another important aspect is to set clear boundaries and expectations for the relationship. This includes establishing what behaviors are and are not acceptable, as well as discussing what each partner needs from the relationship in order to feel loved, supported, and fulfilled.

In addition to communication and boundary-setting, it can also be helpful for both partners to engage in individual therapy or couples therapy. This can provide a safe and supportive space to address any unresolved issues, work through difficult emotions, and develop new strategies for rebuilding the relationship.

Ultimately, rebuilding a relationship after sex addiction requires a willingness to be patient, compassionate, and committed to the process. It may not be easy, but with effort and dedication, it is possible to create a strong, healthy, and fulfilling relationship.

Developing Healthy Sexuality

Developing healthy sexuality is an important aspect of recovery from sex addiction. Sex addiction can cause individuals to lose touch with their own sexual desires and boundaries, leading to unhealthy behaviors and damaging relationships. Learning to establish healthy sexual boundaries and communicate effectively about sexual needs and desires is crucial in developing a healthy sexuality.

One approach to developing healthy sexuality is through therapy. Sex addiction therapy can help individuals explore their own sexual desires, identify and work through any underlying issues or trauma that may be contributing to their addiction, and develop a healthy relationship with sex.

Another approach to developing healthy sexuality is through education and self-exploration. This may include reading about healthy sexuality, attending workshops or classes, and experimenting with different sexual practices in a safe and consensual manner.

Developing healthy sexuality also involves cultivating self-awareness and mindfulness. By becoming more attuned to their own physical and emotional responses, individuals can better understand their own sexual needs and boundaries, and communicate them effectively to partners.

Ultimately, developing healthy sexuality requires a willingness to explore, communicate, and set boundaries. With the right tools and support, individuals can rebuild a healthy relationship with sex and intimacy after sex addiction.

Maintaining Long-Term Recovery

Maintaining long-term recovery from sex addiction requires ongoing effort and commitment. Some strategies that can be helpful include:

1. **Continuing therapy:** It is important to continue attending therapy even after initial treatment is completed. This can help individuals stay accountable and address any ongoing challenges that may arise.

2. **Building a support network:** Having a network of supportive friends, family, and peers who understand the challenges of sex addiction can be invaluable. Joining support groups such as Sex Addicts Anonymous or seeking out a sponsor can also be helpful.

3. **Developing healthy coping mechanisms:** Identifying and developing healthy coping mechanisms is important for maintaining recovery. This might include activities such as exercise, mindfulness practices, or creative outlets.

4. **Practicing self-care:** Prioritizing self-care activities such as getting enough sleep, eating well, and engaging in relaxing activities can help individuals maintain their overall health and well-being.

5. **Setting goals and milestones:** Setting goals and milestones for recovery can provide motivation and a sense of accomplishment. This might include working towards specific achievements in therapy, or setting goals for rebuilding relationships or improving personal finances.

By staying committed to these strategies, individuals can maintain their recovery and live a fulfilling life beyond sex addiction.

Conclusion

In conclusion, sex addiction is a complex issue that can have significant impacts on an individual's emotional, physical, and interpersonal well-being. While the causes of sex addiction are multifaceted, treatment options are available to help individuals recover and maintain long-term sobriety. Successful treatment often involves addressing underlying psychological factors such as trauma, shame, and attachment issues, as well as developing healthy coping mechanisms, improving emotional regulation, and rebuilding relationships. With the right support and resources, individuals with sex addiction can achieve a fulfilling and healthy life beyond recovery.

The Future of Sex Addiction Treatment and Research

Sex addiction is a complex and challenging issue that requires a multidisciplinary approach for successful treatment and recovery. In recent years, there has been a growing recognition of the importance of addressing the underlying psychological factors, such as trauma, shame, and attachment issues, in the treatment of sex addiction. There has also been a shift towards a more holistic approach that focuses on rebuilding relationships and developing healthy sexuality.

As research on sex addiction continues to evolve, it is likely that new treatments and interventions will be developed to improve outcomes for individuals struggling with this condition. It is also important to continue to reduce the stigma associated with sex addiction and to promote awareness and education around this issue.

Ultimately, the goal of sex addiction treatment is to help individuals achieve long-term recovery and to live fulfilling lives free from the negative consequences of their addiction. With the right support, resources, and commitment, it is possible to overcome sex addiction and to build a brighter future.

Final Thoughts and Reflections

"Understanding and Treating Sex Addiction" is a comprehensive guide that explores the complex nature of sex addiction and provides insight into its development, impact, and treatment. The book covers a range of topics, including the neurological and psychological factors that contribute to sex addiction, the emotional and physical consequences of sex addiction, and strategies for recovery and rebuilding relationships. It also emphasizes the importance of addressing underlying issues, such as trauma, attachment styles, and shame, in the treatment of sex addiction. Overall, the book aims to provide a better understanding of sex addiction and to help individuals who are struggling with this issue to achieve lasting recovery and healthy sexuality.

Printed in Great Britain
by Amazon